Air Fryer Delights
An Unmissable Recipe Collection for Your Air Fryer Meals

Kira Hamm

TABLE OF CONTENT

medical or professional advice. The content within this book has been derived from various sources. Please consult a licensed professional before attempting any techniques outlined in this book.

By reading this document, the reader agrees that under no circumstances is the author responsible for any losses, direct or indirect, which are incurred as a result of the use of information contained within this document, including, but not limited to, — errors, omissions, or inaccuracies.

Brussels Sprout with Tomatoes Mix

Preparation Time 10 minutes

Cooking Time:10 minutes

Servings: 3

Ingredients:

- 6 halved cherry tomatoes
- 1 tbsp of olive oil
- 1 pound of Brussel sprouts
- Black pepper and salt
- 1/4 cup of chopped green onions

Directions:

1. Sprinkle pepper and salt on the Brussels sprout.
2. Place it on the Power XL Air Fryer Grill pan.
3. Set the Power XL Air Fryer Grill to air fry function.
4. Cook for 10 minutes at 3500F.
5. Place the cooked sprout in a bowl, add pepper, green onion, salt, olive oil, and cherry tomatoes.
6. Mix well and serve immediately

7. Serving Suggestions: serve with tomato mix or ketchup
8. Directions: & Cooking Tips: trim the Brussels sprout

Nutrition: Calories: 57kcal, Fat: 1g, Carb: 12g, Proteins: 5g

Cheesy Brussels Sprout

Preparation Time 10 minutes

Cooking Time:8 minutes

Servings: 3

Ingredients:

- 1 lemon juice
- 2 tbsp of butter
- 1 pound of Brussel sprout
- 3 tbsp of grated parmesan
- Black pepper and salt

Directions:

1. Place the Brussel sprout on the Power XL Air Fryer Grill pan.
2. Set the Power XL Air Fryer Grill to air fry function.
3. Cook for 8 minutes at 3500F.
4. Heat butter in a pan over medium heat, add pepper, lemon juice, and salt.
5. Add Brussel sprout and parmesan.
6. Serve immediately.
7. Serving Suggestions: serve with mint chutney

8. Directions: & Cooking Tips: rinse the
   Brussel sprout well

Nutrition: Calories: 75kcal, Fat: 5g, Carb: 8g,
Proteins: 6g

Spicy Cabbage

Preparation Time 10 minutes

Cooking Time:8 minutes

Servings: 5

Ingredients:

- 1 grated carrot
- 1/2 tsp of cayenne pepper
- 1/4 cup of apple cider vinegar
- 1 cabbage
- 1 tsp of red pepper flakes
- 1 tbsp of sesame seed oil
- 1/4 cups of apple juice

Directions:

1. Put carrot, cayenne, cabbage, and oil on the Power XL Air Fryer Grill pan.
2. Add vinegar, pepper flakes, and apple juice.
3. Set the Power XL Air Fryer Grill to air fry function.
4. Cook for 8 minutes at 3500F
5. Serve immediately
6. Serving Suggestions: Serve with maple syrup

7. Directions: & Cooking Tips: cut the cabbage into 8 wedges

Nutrition: Calories: 25kcal, Fat: 0g, Carb: 6g, Proteins: 2g

Sweet Baby Carrots

Preparation Time 15 minutes

Cooking Time:10 minutes

Serving: 4

Ingredients:

- 1 tbsp of brown sugar
- 2 cups of baby carrots
- 1/2 tbsp. of melted butter
- Black pepper and salt

Directions:

1. Mix butter, sugar, pepper, carrot, and salt in a bowl.
2. Transfer the mix to the Power XL Air Fryer Grill pan
3. Set the Power XL Air Fryer Grill to air fry function.
4. Cook for 10 minutes at 3500F
5. Serve immediately
6. Serving Suggestions: Serve with maple syrup

Nutrition: Calories: 77kcal, Fat: 3g, Carb: 15g, Proteins: 3g

Zucchini Mix and Herbed Eggplant

Preparation Time 10 minutes

Cooking Time:8 minutes

Servings: 3

Ingredients:

- 1 tsp of dried thyme
- 3 tbsp of olive oil
- 1 eggplant
- 2 tbsp of lemon juice
- 1 tsp of dried oregano
- 3 cubed zucchinis
- Black pepper and salt

Directions:

1. Place the eggplants on the Power XL Air Fryer Grill pan, add thyme, zucchinis, olive oil, salt.
2. Add pepper, oregano, and lemon juice.
3. Set the Power XL Air Fryer Grill to air fry function.
4. Cook for 8 minutes at 3600F
5. Serve immediately

Nutrition: Calories: 55kcal, Fat: 1g, Carb: 13g,

Proteins: 3g

Sweet Potato Toast

Preparation Time: 15 minutes

Cooking Time: 10 minutes

Servings: 2

Ingredients:

- 1 large sweet potato, cut
- Avocado/guacamole
- Hummus
- Radish/Tomato (optional)
- Salt & Pepper
- Lemon slice

Directions:

1. Toast the potatoes in the Power XL Air Fryer Grill for 10 minutes on each side.
2. Spread mashed avocado, add seasoning, top it with radish slices and squeeze a lime over it.
3. Or, spread hummus, seasoning, and your choice of greens.

Nutrition: Calories: 114 kcal, Carbs: 13g, Protein: 2g, Fat: 7g.

Stuffed Portabella Mushroom

Preparation Time: 20 minutes

Cooking Time: 15 minutes

Servings: 2

Ingredients:

- 2 large portabella mushrooms
- Breadcrumbs
- Nutritional yeast (gives a cheesy, savory flavor)
- 1 cup tofu ricotta
- 1/2 cup canned marinara sauce
- 1 cup spinach
- 1/2 tsp. garlic powder
- 1 tsp. dry basil & 1 tsp. dry thyme
- Salt & pepper

Directions:

1. Make ricotta with tofu, lemon juice, nutritional yeast, salt, and pepper. Mix the tofu ricotta, spinach, thyme, basil, marinara sauce, and seasoning.
2. Brush marinara sauce on each mushroom and stuff the filling. Top it with

breadcrumbs, nutritional yeast, and some olive oil.

3. Bake for 15 minutes at 2300C or 4500F in your Power XL Air Fryer Grill.

Nutrition: Calories: 275kcal, Carbs: 10.4g, Protein: 23.0g, Fat: 19.5g.

Pumpkin Quesadillas

Preparation Time: 10 minutes

Cooking Time: 5minutes

Servings: 3

Ingredients:

- 1/2 canned pumpkin (pure)
- 2 gluten-free tortillas
- 1/2 cup refried beans
- 1-2 tbsp. nutritional yeast
- 1 tsp. onion powder
- 1 tsp. garlic powder
- Pinch of cayenne
- Salt & pepper

Directions:

1. Mix the pumpkin with nutritional yeast, onion powder, garlic powder, cayenne, salt, and pepper.
2. Spread the pumpkin paste mixture in one tortilla and the refried beans in another.
3. Sandwich them together and toast in the Power XL Air Fryer Grill for 5 minutes

Nutrition: Calories: 282kcal, Carbs: 37g, Protein:

13g, Fat: 10g.

Toasted-Baked Tofu cubes

Preparation Time: 10 minutes

Cooking Time: 30 minutes

Servings: 2

Ingredients:

- 1/2 block of tofu, cubed
- 1 tbsp. olive oil
- 1 tbsp. nutritional yeast
- 1 tbsp. flour
- 1/4 tsp. black pepper
- 1 tsp. sea salt
- 1/2 tsp. garlic powder

Directions:

1. Combine all the Ingredients: with tofu
2. Preheat the Power XL Air Fryer Grill at 2300C or 4000F.
3. Bake tofu on a lined baking tray for 15-30 minutes, turn it around every 10 minutes.

Nutrition: Calories: 100kcal, Carbs: 5g, Protein: 8g, Fat 6g.

Stuffed Squash

Preparation Time: 40 minutes

Cooking Time: 15 minutes

Servings: 4

Ingredients:

- Acorn squash, halved and deseeded
- 2 cups cooked quinoa
- 1/2 edamame (shelled)
- 1/2 corn kernels
- 1/4 cranberries
- Some scallions, basil, and mint (thinly sliced)
- 2 tbsp. Olive oil
- Salt and pepper
- Lemon juice

Directions:

1. Brush squash pieces with olive oil, salt, and pepper.
2. Bake it at 1760C or 3500F for 35 minutes in the Power XL Air Fryer Grill.
3. Directions: are the filling by mixing all the remaining ingredients. Stuff baked squash

with filling and bake for   another 15 minutes.

Nutrition: Calories: 272kcal, Carbs: 45g, Protein: 7g, Fat 9g.

Sriracha Roasted Potatoes

Preparation Time:30 minutes

Cooking Time: 30 minutes

Servings: 3

Ingredients:

- 3 potatoes, diced
- 2-3 tsp. sriracha
- 1/4 garlic powder
- Salt & pepper
- Olive oil
- Chopped fresh parsley

Directions:

1. Combine the potatoes with the remaining ingredients.
2. Preheat the Power XL Air Fryer Grill at 2300C or 4500F.
3. Line the pan with olive oil and spread the coated potatoes. Sprinkle parsley.
4. Bake for 30 minutes.

Nutrition: Calories 147kcal, Carbs: 24.4, Protein: 3g, Fat 4.7g.

Brussel Sprouts, Mango, Avocado Salsa Tacos

Preparation Time: 25 minutes

Cooking Time: 15 minutes

Servings: 4

Ingredients:

- 4 taco shells
- 8 ounces brussels sprouts, diced
- Half a mango, diced
- Half of an avocado, diced
- 1/2 cup black beans, cooked
- 2 tbsp. onions, chopped
- 1/4 cup cilantro, chopped
- 1 tbsp. jalapeno, chopped
- Lime juice
- Olive oil
- 1 tbsp. taco seasoning
- Salt & Pepper

Directions:

1. Preheat the Power XL Air Fryer Grill at 2300C or 4000F.
2. Mix the sprouts with taco seasoning, olive oil and salt and pepper on the pan.

3. Roast for 15 mins. Turn every 5 mins.

4. To make the salsa, combine the mango, avocado, black beans, lime juice, cilantro, onion, jalapeno, salt, and pepper.

5. Cook taco shells and fill it with the sprouts and salsa.

Nutrition: Calories 407kcal, Carbs: 63.20g, Protein: 11.4g, Fat: 13.9g.

Spaghetti Squash Burrito Bowls

Preparation Time:15 minutes

Cooking Time: 45 minutes

Servings: 2

Ingredients:

- 1 small spaghetti squash
- Zucchini, diced
- 1/4 onion, diced
- Bell peppers, diced
- 3/4 cup black beans, cooked
- 1/2 cup corn kernels
- 1/2 cup salsa
- 2 ounces cheese (optional)
- Olive oil
- 1/2 tsp. dried oregano
- 1/4 tsp. ground cumin
- Salt & pepper

Directions:

1. Preheat the Power XL Air Fryer Grill at 2300C or 4250F on bake setting
2. Microwave the squash for 4 minutes and then cut it in half. Scoop out the seeds.

3. Rub oil, salt, and pepper all over the squash and bake it for 45 minutes.
4. Make the filling by stir-frying bell pepper, zucchini, oregano, corn, salt, and pepper for 10 minutes. Add the salsa and black beans.
5. Scrape squash flesh to make spaghetti and toss in the vegetables.
6. Bake them at 1760C or 3500F for 10 minutes and then broil for 1-2 minutes.

Nutrition: Calories: 390kcal, Carbs: 51.4g, Protein: 15.7g, Fat 17.1g.

Baked Oatmeal

This wholesome breakfast is perfect to start your day.

Preparation Time:15 minutes

Cooking Time: 25-35 minutes

Servings: 2

Ingredients:

- 1 cup original oats
- 1 banana
- 1/4 cup pecans
- 1/2 cup milk
- 1 tbsp. flax meal
- 2 tsp. olive oil
- 2 tsp. maple syrup
- 1/2 tsp. baking powder
- 1/2 tsp. ground cinnamon & salt
- 1/2 tsp. vanilla-extract

Directions:

1. Preheat the Power XL Air Fryer Grill at 1760C or 3500F on the baking setting.
2. Make a batter with mashed banana and all the ingredients.

3. Grease a 7x5-inch dish and pour your batter into it. Bake it for 25-35 minutes.

Nutrition: Calories: 235kcal, Carbs: 28.6g, Protein: 4.9g, Fat: 13.2g

Healthy Mixed Vegetables

Preparation Time: 10 minutes

Cooking Time: 10 minutes

Servings: 6

Ingredients:

- 2 cups mushrooms, cut in half
- 2 yellow squash, sliced
- 2 medium zucchinis, sliced
- 3/4 tsp Italian seasoning
- 1/2 onion, sliced
- 1/2 cup olive oil
- 1/2 tsp garlic salt

Directions:

1. Add vegetables and remaining Ingredients into the mixing bowl and toss well.
2. Add vegetables into the air fryer basket and cook at 400 F for 10 minutes. Shake basket halfway through.
3. Serve and enjoy.

Nutrition: Calories 176 Fat 17.3 g Carbohydrates 6.2 g Sugar 3.2 g Protein 2.5 g Cholesterol 0 mg

Easy Roasted Vegetables

Preparation Time:10 minutes

Cooking Time: 18 minutes

Servings:6

Ingredients:

- 1/2 cup mushrooms, sliced
- 1/2 cup zucchini, sliced
- 1/2 cup yellow squash, sliced
- 1/2 cup baby carrots
- 1 cup cauliflower florets
- 1 cup broccoli florets
- 1/4 cup parmesan cheese, grated
- 1 tsp red pepper flakes
- 1 tbsp garlic, minced
- 1 tbsp olive oil
- 1/4 cup balsamic vinegar
- 1 small onion, sliced
- 1 tsp sea salt

Directions:

1. Preheat the cosori air fryer to 400 F.
2. In a large mixing bowl, mix together olive oil, garlic, vinegar, red pepper flakes, pepper, and salt.

3. Add vegetables and toss until well coated.

4. Add vegetables into the air fryer basket and cook for 8 minutes. Shake basket and cook for 8 minutes more.

5. Add parmesan cheese and cook for 2 minutes more.

6. Serve and enjoy.

Nutrition: Calories 59 Fat 3.4 g Carbohydrates 5.3 g Sugar 2 g Protein 2.8 g Cholesterol 3 mg

Easy & Crisp Brussels Sprouts

Preparation Time:10 minutes

Cooking Time: 15 minutes

Servings:4

Ingredients:

- 2 cups Brussels sprouts
- 2 tbsp everything bagel seasoning
- 1/4 cup almonds, crushed
- 1/4 cup parmesan cheese, grated
- 2 tbsp olive oil
- Salt

Directions:

1. Add Brussels sprouts into the saucepan with 2 cups of water. Cover and cook for 8-10 minutes.
2. Drain well and allow to cool completely. Sliced each Brussels sprouts in half.
3. Add Brussels sprouts and remaining Ingredients into the mixing bowl and toss to coat.

4. Add Brussels sprouts mixture into the air fryer basket and cook at 375 F for 12-15 minutes.
5. Serve and enjoy.

Nutrition: Calories 144 Fat 11.5 g Carbohydrates 7.6 g Sugar 1.4 g Protein 5.1 g Cholesterol 4 mg

Garlic Green Beans

Preparation Time:10 minutes

Cooking Time: 8 minutes

Servings:4

Ingredients:

- 1 lb. fresh green beans, trimmed
- 1 tsp garlic powder
- 1 tbsp olive oil
- Pepper
- Salt

Directions:

1. Drizzle green beans with oil and season with garlic powder, pepper, and salt.
2. Place green beans into the air fryer basket and cook at 370 F for 8 minutes. Toss halfway through.
3. Serve and enjoy.

Nutrition: Calories 68 Fat 3.7 g Carbohydrates 8.6 g Sugar 1.8 g Protein 2.2 g Cholesterol 0 mg

Simple Vegan Broccoli

Preparation Time:10 minutes

Cooking Time: 5 minutes

Servings:2

Ingredients:

- 4 cups broccoli florets
- 1 tbsp nutritional yeast
- 2 tbsp olive oil
- Pepper
- Salt

Directions:

1. In a medium bowl, mix together broccoli, nutritional yeast, oil, pepper, and salt.
2. Add broccoli florets into the air fryer basket and cook at 370 F for 5 minutes.
3. Serve and enjoy.

Nutrition: Calories 158 Fat 14.3 g Carbohydrates 6.3 g Sugar 1 g Protein 4.3 g Cholesterol 0 mg

Sesame Carrots

Preparation Time:10 minutes

Cooking Time: 7 minutes

Servings:4

Ingredients:

- 2 cups carrots, sliced
- 1 tsp sesame seeds
- 1 tbsp scallions, chopped
- 1 tsp garlic, minced
- 1 tbsp soy sauce
- 1 tbsp ginger, minced
- 2 tbsp sesame oil

Directions:

1. In a medium bowl, mix together carrots, garlic, soy sauce, ginger, and sesame oil.
2. Add carrots mixture into the air fryer basket and cook at 375 for 7 minutes. Shake basket halfway through.
3. Garnish with scallions and sesame seeds and serve.

Nutrition: Calories 95 Fat 7.3 g Carbohydrates 7.2 g Sugar 2.9 g Protein 1 g Cholesterol 0 mg

Asparagus with Almonds

Preparation Time:10 minutes

Cooking Time: 5 minutes

Servings:4

Ingredients:

- 12 asparagus spears
- 1/3 cup sliced almonds
- 2 tbsp olive oil
- 2 tbsp balsamic vinegar
- Pepper
- Salt

Directions:

1. Drizzle asparagus spears with oil and vinegar.
2. Arrange asparagus spears into the air fryer basket and season with pepper and salt.
3. Sprinkle sliced almond over asparagus spears.
4. Cook asparagus at 350 F for 5 minutes. Shake basket halfway through.
5. Serve and enjoy.

Nutrition: Calories 122 Fat 11.1 g Carbohydrates 4.6 g Sugar 1.7 g Protein 3.3 g Cholesterol 0 mg

Easy Roasted Carrots

Preparation Time:10 minutes

Cooking Time: 18 minutes

Servings:4

Ingredients:

- 16 oz carrots, peeled and cut into 2-inch chunks
- 1 tsp olive oil
- Pepper
- Salt

Directions:

1. Preheat the cosori air fryer to 360 F.
2. Toss carrots with oil and season with pepper and salt.
3. Add carrots into the air fryer basket and cook for 15-18 minutes. Shake basket 3-4 Times.
4. Serve and enjoy.

Nutrition: Calories 57 Fat 1.2 g Carbohydrates 11.2 g Sugar 5.6 g Protein 0.9 g Cholesterol 0 mg

Asian Broccoli

Preparation Time:10 minutes

Cooking Time: 20 minutes

Servings:4

Ingredients:

- 1 lb. broccoli florets
- 1 tsp rice vinegar
- 2 tsp sriracha
- 2 tbsp soy sauce
- 1 tbsp garlic, minced
- 1 1/2 tbsp sesame oil
- Salt

Directions:

1. Toss broccoli florets with garlic, sesame oil, and salt.
2. Add broccoli florets into the air fryer basket and cook at 400 F for 15-20 minutes. Shake basket halfway through.
3. In a mixing bowl, mix together rice vinegar, sriracha, and soy sauce. Add broccoli and toss well.
4. Serve and enjoy.

Nutrition: Calories 94 Fat 5.5 g Carbohydrates 9.3 g

Sugar 2.1 g Protein 3.8 g Cholesterol 0 mg

Healthy Squash & Zucchini

Preparation Time:10 minutes

Cooking Time: 25 minutes

Servings:4

Ingredients:

- 1 lb. zucchini, cut into 1/2-inch half-moons
- 1 lb. yellow squash, cut into 1/2-inch half-moons
- 1 tbsp olive oil
- Pepper
- Salt

Directions:

1. In a mixing bowl, add zucchini, squash, oil, pepper, and salt and toss well.
2. Add zucchini and squash mixture into the air fryer basket and cook at 400 F for 20 minutes. Shake basket halfway through.
3. Shake basket well and cook for 5 minutes more.
4. Serve and enjoy.

Nutrition: Calories 66 Fat 3.9 g Carbohydrates 7.6 g Sugar 3.9 g Protein 2.7 g Cholesterol 0 mg

Crunchy Fried Cabbage

Preparation Time:10 minutes

Cooking Time: 10 minutes

Servings:2

Ingredients:

- 1/2 cabbage head, sliced into 2-inch slices
- 1 tbsp olive oil
- Pepper
- Salt

Directions:

1. Drizzle cabbage with olive oil and season with pepper and salt.
2. Add cabbage slices into the air fryer basket and cook at 375 F for 5 minutes.
3. Toss cabbage well and cook for 5 minutes more.
4. Serve and enjoy.

Nutrition: Calories 105 Fat 7.2 g Carbohydrates 10.4 g Sugar 5.7 g Protein 2.3 g Cholesterol 0 mg

Quick Vegetable Kebabs

Preparation Time:10 minutes

Cooking Time: 10 minutes

Servings:4

Ingredients:

- 2 bell peppers, cut into 1-inch pieces
- 1/2 onion, cut into 1-inch pieces
- 1 zucchini, cut into 1-inch pieces
- 1 eggplant, cut into 1-inch pieces
- Pepper
- Salt

Directions:

1. Thread vegetables onto the skewers and spray them with cooking spray. Season with pepper and salt.
2. Preheat the cosori air fryer to 390 F.
3. Place skewers into the air fryer basket and cooks for 10 minutes. Turn halfway through.
4. Serve and enjoy.

Nutrition: Calories 48 Fat 0.3 g Carbohydrates 11.2 g Sugar 5.9 g Protein 2.1 g Cholesterol 0 mg

Easy Soy Garlic Mushrooms

Preparation Time:10 minutes

Cooking Time: 12 minutes

Servings:2

Ingredients:

- 8 oz mushrooms, cleaned
- 1 tbsp fresh parsley, chopped
- 1 tsp soy sauce
- 1/2 tsp garlic powder
- 1 tbsp olive oil
- Pepper
- Salt

Directions:

1. Toss mushrooms with soy sauce, garlic powder, oil, pepper, and salt.
2. Add mushrooms into the air fryer basket and cook at 380 F for 10-12 minutes.
3. Garnish with parsley and serve.

Nutrition: Calories 89 Fat 7.4 g Carbohydrates 4.6 g Sugar 2.2 g Protein 3.9 g Cholesterol 0 mg

Spicy Edamame

Preparation Time:10 minutes

Cooking Time: 18 minutes

Servings:4

Ingredients:

- 16 oz frozen edamame in shell, defrosted
- 1 lemon juice
- 1 lemon zest
- 1 tbsp garlic, sliced
- 2 tsp olive oil
- 1/2 tsp chili powder
- 1/2 tsp paprika
- Salt

Directions:

1. Toss edamame with lemon zest, garlic, oil, chili powder, paprika, and salt.
2. Add edamame into the air fryer basket and cook at 400 F for 18 minutes. Shake basket twice.
3. Drizzle lemon juice over edamame and serve.

Nutrition: Calories 172 Fat 8.5 g Carbohydrates 12.2 g Sugar 2.7 g Protein 12.3 g Cholesterol 0 mg

Balsamic Mushrooms

Preparation Time:10 minutes

Cooking Time: 8 minutes

Servings:3

Ingredients:

- 8 oz mushrooms
- 1 tsp fresh parsley, chopped
- 2 tsp balsamic vinegar
- 1/2 tsp granulated garlic
- 1 tsp olive oil
- Pepper
- Salt

Directions:

1. Toss mushrooms with garlic, oil, pepper, and salt.
2. Add mushrooms into the air fryer basket and cook at 375 F for 8 minutes. Toss halfway through.
3. Toss mushrooms with parsley and balsamic vinegar.
4. Serve and enjoy.

Nutrition: Calories 32 Fat 1.8 g Carbohydrates 2.9 g Sugar 1.4 g Protein 2.5 g Cholesterol 0 mg

Mediterranean Vegetables

Preparation Time:10 minutes

Cooking Time: 15 minutes

Servings:2

Ingredients:

- 6 cherry tomatoes, cut in half
- 1 eggplant, diced
- 1 zucchini, diced
- 1 green bell pepper, diced
- 1 tsp thyme
- 1 tsp oregano
- Pepper
- Salt

Directions:

1. In a bowl, toss eggplant, zucchini, bell pepper, thyme, oregano, pepper, and salt.
2. Add vegetable mixture into the air fryer basket and cook at 360 F for 12 minutes.
3. Add cherry tomatoes and shake basket well and cook for 3 minutes more.
4. Serve and enjoy.

Nutrition: Calories 61 Fat 0.3 g Carbohydrates 13.8 g Sugar 7.6 g Protein 2.8 g Cholesterol 0 mg

Simple Roasted Okra

Preparation Time:10 minutes

Cooking Time: 12 minutes

Servings:1

Ingredients:

- 1/2 lb. okra, trimmed and sliced
- 1 tsp olive oil
- Pepper
- Salt

Directions:

1. Preheat the cosori air fryer to 350 F.
2. Mix together okra, oil, pepper, and salt.
3. Add okra into the air fryer basket and cook for 10 minutes. Toss halfway through.
4. Toss well and cook for 2 minutes more.
5. Serve and enjoy.

Nutrition: Calories 176 Fat 17.3 g Carbohydrates 6.2 g Sugar 3.2 g Protein 2.5 g Cholesterol 0 mg

Air Fried Vegetables

Preparation Time:10 minutes

Cooking Time: 8 minutes

Servings:3

Ingredients:

- 2 tablespoons extra virgin olive oil
- 1 tablespoon minced garlic
- 1 large shallot, sliced
- 1 cup mushrooms, sliced
- 1 cup broccoli florets
- 1 cup artichoke hearts
- 1 bunch asparagus, sliced into 3-inch pieces
- 1 cup baby peas
- 1 cup cherry tomatoes, halved
- 1/2 teaspoon sea salt
- Vinaigrette
- 3 tablespoons white wine vinegar
- 6 tablespoons extra-virgin olive oil
- 1/2 teaspoon sea salt
- 1 teaspoon ground oregano
- handful fresh parsley, chopped

Directions:

1. Add oil to the pan of your air fryer toast oven set over medium heat. Stir in garlic and shallots and air fry for about 2 minutes.
2. Stir in mushrooms for about 3 minutes or until golden.
3. Stir in broccoli, artichokes, and asparagus and continue cooking for 3 more minutes. Stir in peas, tomatoes and salt and transfer to the air fryer toast oven and cook for 5-8 more minutes.
4. Directions: are vinaigrette: mix together vinegar, oil, salt, oregano and parsley in a bowl until well combined.
5. Serve the air fried vegetable in a serving bowl and drizzle with vinaigrette. Toss to combine and serve.

Nutrition: Calories: 293 kcal, Carbs: 14.6 g, Fat: 27 g, Protein: 25 g.

Air Broiled Mushrooms

Preparation Time:10 minutes

Cooking Time: 10 minutes

Servings: 4

Ingredients:

- 2 cups shiitake mushrooms
- 1 tablespoon balsamic vinegar
- 1/4 cup extra virgin olive oil
- 1-2 garlic cloves, minced
- A handful of parsley
- 1 teaspoon salt

Directions:

1. Rinse the mushroom and pat dry; put in a foil and drizzle with balsamic vinegar and extra virgin olive oil.
2. Sprinkle the mushroom with garlic, parsley, and salt.
3. Broil for about 10 minutes in your air fryer toast oven at 350 degrees F or until tender and cooked through. Serve warm.

Nutrition: Calories: 260 kcal, Carbs: 11 g, Fat: 19.1 g, Protein: 22 g.

Hydrated Potato Wedges

Preparation Time:5 minutes

Cooking Time: 30 minutes

Servings: 5

Ingredients:

- 2 medium Russet potatoes, diced into wedges
- 1 1/2 tablespoons olive oil
- 1/2 teaspoon chili powder
- 1/2 teaspoon parsley
- 1/2 teaspoon paprika
- 1/8 teaspoon black pepper
- 1/2 teaspoon sea salt

Directions:

1. In a large bowl, mix potato wedges, olive oil, chili, parsley, paprika, salt and pepper until the potatoes are well coated.
2. Transfer half of the potatoes to a fryer basket and hydrate for 20 minutes.
3. Repeat with the remaining wedges. Serve hot with chilled orange juice.

Nutrition: Calories: 129 kcal, Carbs: 10 g, Fat: 5.3 g, Protein: 2.3 g.

Crispy Baked Tofu

Preparation Time:15 minutes

Cooking Time: 20 minutes

Servings: 4

Ingredients:

- 1 cup whole wheat flour
- 1 package (16-ounce) extra firm tofu, chopped into 8 slices
- 3/4 cup raw cashews
- 2 cups pretzel sticks
- 1 tbsp. extra virgin olive oil
- 2 tsp. chili powder
- 1 cup unsweetened almond milk
- 2 tsp. garlic powder
- 2 tsp. onion powder
- 1 tsp. lemon pepper
- 1/4 tsp. black pepper
- 1/2 tsp. sea salt

Directions:

1. Preheat your air fryer toast oven to 400 degrees F.
2. Line a baking sheet with baking paper and set aside.

3. In a food processor, pulse together cashews and pretzel stick until coarsely ground.
4. Combine garlic, onion, chili powder, lemon pepper, and salt in a small bowl.
5. In a large bowl, combine half of the spice mixture and flour.
6. Add almond milk to a separate bowl.
7. In another bowl, combine cashew mixture, salt, pepper and olive oil; mix well.
8. Sprinkle tofu slices with the remaining half of the spice mixture and coat each with the flour and then dip in almond mil; coat with the cashew mixture and bake for about 18 minutes or until golden brown.
9. Serve the baked tofu with favorite vegan salad.

Nutrition: Calories: 332 kcal, Carbs: 23.3 g, Fat: 8.8 g, Protein: 12.9 g.

Spiced Tempeh

Preparation Time: 15 minutes

Cooking Time: 20 minutes

Servings: 4

Ingredients:

- Tempeh Bits:
- 1/4 cup vegetable oil
- 8 oz. tempeh
- 1 tsp. lemon pepper
- 1 tsp. chili powder
- 2 tsp. sweet paprika
- 2 tsp. garlic powder
- 2 tsp. onion powder
- 1/4 tsp. sea salt
- 1/8 tsp. cayenne pepper or more to taste
- Salad:
- 15.5 oz. can chickpeas
- 1 lb. chopped kale
- 1 cup shredded carrots
- 2 tbsp. sesame seeds, toasted
- Dressing:
- 1 tbsp. fresh grated ginger
- 2 tbsp. toasted sesame oil

- 1/4 cup low sodium soy sauce
- 1/3 cup seasoned rice vinegar

Directions:

1. Blanch kale in a pot of salted boiling water for about 30 seconds and immediately run under cold water; drain and squeeze out excess water. Set aside.
2. Preheat your air fryer toast oven to 425 degrees F.
3. In a small bowl, combine all the spices for tempeh.
4. Add oil to a separate bowl. Slice tempeh into thin pieces.
5. Dip each tempeh slice into the oil and arrange them on a paper-lined baking sheet; generously sprinkle with the spices until well covered and bake for about 20 minutes or until crispy and golden brown then remove from air fryer toast oven. In a large bowl, combine all the salad ingredients and set aside.
6. In a jar, combine all the dressing Ingredients: close and shake until well

blended; pour the dressing over salad and toss to coat well.

7. Crumble the crispy tempeh on top of the salad to serve. Enjoy!

Nutrition: Calories: 308 kcal, Carbs: 19.2 g, Fat: 7.3 g, Protein: 9.8 g.

Steamed Broccoli

Preparation Time:8 minutes

Cooking Time: 3 minutes

Servings: 2

Ingredients:

- 1 pound broccoli florets
- 1-1/2 cups water
- Salt and pepper to taste
- I tsp. extra virgin olive oil

Directions:

1. Add water to the bottom of your air fryer toast oven and set the basket on top.
2. Toss the broccoli florets with, salt pepper and olive oil until evenly combined then transfer to the basket of your air fryer toast oven.
3. Select keep warm for 10 minutes.
4. Remove the basket and serve the broccoli.

Nutrition: Calories: 160 kcal, Carbs: 6.1 g, Fat: 12 g, Protein: 13 g.

Air Fried Brussel Sprouts

Preparation Time:10 minutes

Cooking Time: 10 minutes

Servings: 4

Ingredients:

- 2-pound Brussels sprouts, halved
- 1 tbsp. chopped almonds
- 1 tbsp. rice vinegar
- 2 tbsp. sriracha sauce
- 1/4 cup gluten free soy sauce
- 2 tbsp. sesame oil
- 1/2 tbsp. cayenne pepper
- 1 tbsp. smoked paprika
- 1 tsp. onion powder
- 2 tsp. garlic powder
- 1 tsp. red pepper flakes
- Salt and pepper

Directions:

1. Preheat your air fryer toast oven to 370 degrees F.
2. Meanwhile place your air fryer toast oven's pan on medium heat and cook the almonds

for 3 minutes then add in all the remaining ingredients.

3. Place the pan in the air fryer toast oven and air fry for 8-10 minutes or until done to desire.

4. Serve hot over a bed of steamed rice.

5. Enjoy!

Nutrition: Calories: 216 kcal, Carbs: 8.8 g, Fat: 18 g, Protein: 18g.

Hydrated Kale Chips

Preparation Time: 5 minutes

Cooking Time: 5 minutes

Servings: 2

Ingredients:

1. 4 cups loosely packed kale, stemmed
2. 2 teaspoons ranch Seasoning
3. 2 tablespoons olive oil
4. 1 tablespoon nutritional yeast
5. 1/4 teaspoon salt

Directions:

1. In a bowl, toss together kale pieces, oil, nutritional yeast, ranch seasoning, and salt until well coated.
2. Transfer to a fryer basket and hydrate for 15 minutes, shaking halfway through cooking.
3. Serve right away!

Nutrition: Calories: 103 kcal, Carbs: 8.2 g, Fat: 7.1 g, Protein: 3.2 g.

Parmesan Asparagus

Preparation Time:10 minutes

Cooking Time: 5 minutes

Servings:2

Ingredients:

- 1 egg, lightly beaten
- 10 asparagus spears, trimmed and cut woody ends
- 1 tbsp heavy cream
- 1/3 cup parmesan cheese, grated
- 1/3 cup almond flour
- 1/2 tsp paprika

Directions:

1. Spray air fryer basket with cooking spray.
2. In a shallow dish, whisk together egg and cream until well mix.
3. In a separate dish, mix together almond flour, parmesan cheese, paprika, and salt.
4. Dip asparagus spear into the egg mixture then coat with almond flour mixture.
5. Place coated asparagus into the air fryer basket and cook at 350 F for 5 minutes.

Nutrition: Calories 166 Fat 11.3 g Carbohydrates 7 g

Sugar 2.7 g Protein 12.3 g Cholesterol 105 mg

Greek Vegetables

Preparation Time: 10 minutes

Cooking Time: 20 minutes

Servings: 4

Ingredients:

- 1 carrot, sliced
- 1 parsnip, sliced
- 1 green bell pepper, chopped
- 1 courgette, chopped
- 1/4 cup cherry tomatoes, cut in half
- 6 tbsp olive oil
- 2 tsp garlic puree
- 1 tsp mustard
- 1 tsp mixed herbs
- Pepper
- Salt

Directions:

1. Add cherry tomatoes, carrot, parsnip, bell pepper, and courgette into the air fryer basket.
2. Drizzle olive oil over vegetables and cook at 350 F for 15 minutes.

3. In a mixing bowl, mix together the remaining ingredients. Add vegetables into the mixing bowl and toss well.
4. Return vegetables to the air fryer basket and cook at 400 F for 5 minutes more.
5. Serve and enjoy.

Nutrition: Calories 66 Fat 1.5 g Carbohydrates 12.7 g Sugar 5.3 g Protein 1.8 g Cholesterol 1 mg

Lemon Garlic Cauliflower

Preparation Time:10 minutes

Cooking Time: 10 minutes

Servings:2

Ingredients:

- 3 cups cauliflower
- 1 tbsp fresh parsley, chopped
- 1/2 tsp lemon juice
- 1 tbsp pine nuts
- 1/2 tsp dried oregano
- 1 1/2 tsp olive oil
- Pepper
- Salt

Directions:

1. Add cauliflower, oregano, oil, pepper, and salt into the mixing bowl and toss well.
2. Add cauliflower into the air fryer basket and cook at 375 F for 10 minutes.
3. Transfer cauliflower into the serving bowl. Add pine nuts, parsley, and lemon juice and toss well.
4. Serve and enjoy.

Nutrition: Calories 99 Fat 6.7 g Carbohydrates 8.9 g

Sugar 3.8 g Protein 3.7 g Cholesterol 0 mg

Balsamic Brussels Sprouts

Preparation Time: 10 minutes

Cooking Time: 20 minutes

Servings: 4

Ingredients:

- 1 lb. brussels sprouts, remove ends and cut in half
- 1 tbsp balsamic vinegar
- 2 tbsp olive oil
- Pepper
- Salt

Directions:

1. Add brussels sprouts, vinegar, oil, pepper, and salt into the mixing bowl and toss well.
2. Add brussels sprouts into the air fryer basket and cook at 360 F for 15-20 minutes. Toss halfway through.
3. Serve and enjoy.

Nutrition: Calories 110 Fat 7.4 g Carbohydrates 10.4 g Sugar 2.5 g Protein 3.9 g Cholesterol 0 mg

Flavorful Butternut Squash

Preparation Time:10 minutes

Cooking Time: 15 minutes

Servings:4

Ingredients:

- 4 cups butternut squash, cut into 1-inch pieces
- 1 tsp Chinese five-spice powder
- 1 tbsp truvia
- 2 tbsp olive oil

Directions:

1. Add butternut squash and remaining Ingredients into the mixing bowl and mix well.
2. Add butternut squash into the air fryer basket and cook at 400 F for 15 minutes. Shake basket halfway through.
3. Serve and enjoy.

Nutrition: Calories 83 Fat 7.1 g Carbohydrates 6.7 g Sugar 2.2 g Protein 0.6 g Cholesterol 0 mg

Crispy Green Beans

Preparation Time:10 minutes

Cooking Time: 10 minutes

Servings:4

Ingredients:

- 2 cups green beans, ends trimmed
- 2 tbsp parmesan cheese, shredded
- 1 tbsp fresh lemon juice
- 1 tsp Italian seasoning
- 2 tsp olive oil
- 1/4 tsp salt

Directions:

1. Preheat the cosori air fryer to 400 F.
2. Brush green beans with olive oil and season with Italian seasoning and salt.
3. Place green beans into the air fryer basket and cook for 8-10 minutes. Shake basket 2-3 Times.
4. Transfer green beans on a serving plate.
5. Pour lemon juice over beans and sprinkle shredded cheese on top of beans.
6. Serve and enjoy.

Nutrition: Calories 64 Fat 4.3 g Carbohydrates 4.4 g

Sugar 1 g Protein 3.3 g Cholesterol 6 mg

Roasted Zucchini

Preparation Time:10 minutes

Cooking Time: 10 minutes

Servings:4

Ingredients:

- 2 medium zucchinis, cut into 1-inch slices
- 1 tsp lemon zest
- 1 tbsp olive oil
- Pepper
- Salt

Directions:

1. Toss zucchini with lemon zest, oil, pepper, and salt.
2. Arrange zucchini slices into the air fryer basket and cook at 350 F for 10 minutes. Turn halfway through.
3. Serve and enjoy.

Nutrition: Calories 46 Fat 3.7 g Carbohydrates 3.4 g Sugar 1.7 g Protein 1.2 g Cholesterol 0 mg

Air Fried Carrots, Zucchini & Squash

Preparation Time:10 minutes

Cooking Time: 35 minutes

Servings:2

Ingredients:

- 1 lb. yellow squash, cut into 3/4-inch half-moons
- 1 lb. zucchini, cut into 3/4-inch half-moons
- 1/2 lb. carrots, peeled and cut into 1-inch pieces
- 6 tsp olive oil
- 1 tbsp tarragon, chopped
- Pepper
- Salt

Directions:

1. In a bowl, toss carrots with 2 tsp oil. Add carrots into the air fryer basket and cook at 400 F for 5 minutes.
2. In a mixing bowl, toss squash, zucchini, remaining oil, pepper, and salt.

3. Add squash and zucchini mixture into the air fryer basket with carrots and cook for 30 minutes. Shake basket 2-3 Times.

4. Sprinkle with tarragon and serve.

Nutrition: Calories 176 Fat 17.3 g Carbohydrates 6.2 g Sugar 3.2 g Protein 2.5 g Cholesterol 0 mg

Crispy & Spicy Eggplant

Preparation Time:10 minutes

Cooking Time: 20 minutes

Servings:4

Ingredients:

- 1 eggplant, cut into 1-inch pieces
- 1/2 tsp Italian seasoning
- 1 tsp paprika
- 1/2 tsp red pepper
- 1 tsp garlic powder
- 2 tbsp olive oil

Directions:

1. Add eggplant and remaining Ingredients into the bowl and toss well.
2. Spray air fryer basket with cooking spray.
3. Add eggplant into the air fryer basket and cook at 375 F for 20 minutes. Shake basket halfway through.
4. Serve and enjoy.

Nutrition: Calories 99 Fat 7.5 g Carbohydrates 8.7 g Sugar 4.5 g Protein 1.5 g Cholesterol 0 mg

Curried Eggplant Slices

Preparation Time:10 minutes

Cooking Time: 10 minutes

Servings:4

Ingredients:

- 1 large eggplant, cut into 1/2-inch slices
- 1 garlic clove, minced
- 1 tbsp olive oil
- 1/2 tsp curry powder
- 1/8 tsp turmeric
- Salt

Directions:

1. Preheat the cosori air fryer to 300 F.
2. In a small bowl, mix together oil, garlic, curry powder, turmeric, and salt and rub all over eggplant slices.
3. Add eggplant slices into the air fryer basket and cook for 10 minutes or until lightly browned.
4. Serve and enjoy.

Nutrition: Calories 61 Fat 3.8 g Carbohydrates 7.2 g Sugar 3.5 g Protein 1.2 g Cholesterol 0 mg

Spiced Green Beans

Preparation Time:10 minutes

Cooking Time: 10 minutes

Servings:2

Ingredients:

- 2 cups green beans
- 1/8 tsp ground allspice
- 1/4 tsp ground cinnamon
- 1/2 tsp dried oregano
- 2 tbsp olive oil
- 1/4 tsp ground coriander
- 1/4 tsp ground cumin
- 1/8 tsp cayenne pepper
- 1/2 tsp salt

Directions:

1. Add all Ingredients into the medium bowl and toss well.
2. Spray air fryer basket with cooking spray.
3. Add green beans into the air fryer basket and cook at 370 F for 10 minutes. Shake basket halfway through
4. Serve and enjoy.

Nutrition: Calories 158 Fat 14.3 g Carbohydrates 8.6

g Sugar 1.6 g Protein 2.1 g Cholesterol 0 mg

Air Fryer Basil Tomatoes

Preparation Time:10 minutes

Cooking Time: 25 minutes

Servings:4

Ingredients:

- 4 large tomatoes, halved
- 1 garlic clove, minced
- 1 tbsp vinegar
- 1 tbsp olive oil
- 2 tbsp parmesan cheese, grated
- 1/2 tsp fresh parsley, chopped
- 1 tsp fresh basil, minced
- Pepper
- Salt

Directions:

1. Preheat the cosori air fryer to 320 F.
2. In a bowl, mix together oil, basil, garlic, vinegar, pepper, and salt. Add tomatoes and stir to coat.
3. Place tomato halves into the air fryer basket and cook for 20 minutes.
4. Sprinkle parmesan cheese over tomatoes and cook for 5 minutes more.

5. Serve and enjoy.

Nutrition: Calories 87 Fat 5.4 g Carbohydrates 7.7 g Sugar 4.8 g Protein 3.9 g Cholesterol 5 mg

Air Fryer Ratatouille

Preparation Time:10 minutes

Cooking Time: 15 minutes

Servings:6

Ingredients:

- 1 eggplant, diced
- 1 onion, diced
- 3 tomatoes, diced
- 1 red bell pepper, diced
- 1 green bell pepper, diced
- 1 tbsp vinegar
- 2 tbsp olive oil
- 2 tbsp herb de Provence
- 2 garlic cloves, chopped
- Pepper
- Salt

Directions:

1. Preheat the cosori air fryer to 400 F.
2. Add all Ingredients into the bowl and toss well and transfer into the air fryer safe dish.
3. Place dish into the air fryer basket and cook for 15 minutes. Stir halfway through.
4. Serve and enjoy.

Nutrition: Calories 91 Fat 5 g Carbohydrates 11.6 g Sugar 6.4 g Protein 1.9 g Cholesterol 0 mg

Garlicky Cauliflower Florets

Preparation Time:10 minutes

Cooking Time: 20 minutes

Servings:4

Ingredients:

- 5 cups cauliflower florets
- 1/2 tsp cumin powder
- 1/2 tsp ground coriander
- 6 garlic cloves, chopped
- 4 tablespoons olive oil
- 1/2 tsp salt

Directions:

1. Add cauliflower florets and remaining Ingredients into the large mixing bowl and toss well.
2. Add cauliflower florets into the air fryer basket and cook at 400 F for 20 minutes. Shake basket halfway through.
3. Serve and enjoy.

Nutrition: Calories 159 Fat 14.2 g Carbohydrates 8.2 g Sugar 3.1 g Protein 2.8 g Cholesterol 0 mg

Parmesan Brussels Sprouts

Preparation Time:10 minutes

Cooking Time: 12 minutes

Servings:4

Ingredients:

- 1 lb. Brussels sprouts, remove stems and halved
- 1/4 cup parmesan cheese, grated
- 2 tbsp olive oil
- Pepper
- Salt

Directions:

1. Preheat the cosori air fryer to 350 F.
2. In a mixing bowl, toss Brussels sprouts with oil, pepper, and salt.
3. Transfer Brussels sprouts into the air fryer basket and cook for 12 minutes. Shake basket halfway through.
4. Sprinkle with parmesan cheese and serve.

Nutrition: Calories 129 Fat 8.7 g Carbohydrates 10.6 g Sugar 2.5 g Protein 5.9 g Cholesterol 4 mg

Flavorful Tomatoes

Preparation Time:10 minutes

Cooking Time: 15 minutes

Servings:4

Ingredients:

- 4 Roma tomatoes, sliced, remove seeds pithy portion
- 1 tbsp olive oil
- 1/2 tsp dried thyme
- 2 garlic cloves, minced
- Pepper
- Salt

Directions:

1. Preheat the cosori air fryer to 390 F.
2. Toss sliced tomatoes with oil, thyme, garlic, pepper, and salt.
3. Arrange sliced tomatoes into the air fryer basket and cook for 15 minutes.
4. Serve and enjoy.

Nutrition: Calories 55 Fat 3.8 g Carbohydrates 5.4 g Sugar 3.3 g Protein 1.2 g Cholesterol 0 mg

Healthy Roasted Carrots

Preparation Time:10 minutes

Cooking Time: 12 minutes

Servings:4

Ingredients:

- 2 cups carrots, peeled and chopped
- 1 tsp cumin
- 1 tbsp olive oil
- 1/4 fresh coriander, chopped
- Directions:
- Toss carrots with cumin and oil and place them into the air fryer basket.
- Cook at 390 F for 12 minutes.
- Garnish with fresh coriander and serve.

Nutrition: Calories 55 Fat 3.6 g Carbohydrates 5.7 g Sugar 2.7 g Protein 0.6 g Cholesterol 0 mg

Curried Cauliflower with Pine Nuts

Preparation Time:10 minutes

Cooking Time: 10 minutes

Servings:4

Ingredients:

- 1 small cauliflower head, cut into florets
- 2 tbsp olive oil
- 1/4 cup pine nuts, toasted
- 1 tbsp curry powder
- 1/4 tsp salt

Directions:

1. Preheat the cosori air fryer to 350 F.
2. In a mixing bowl, toss cauliflower florets with oil, curry powder, and salt.
3. Add cauliflower florets into the air fryer basket and cook for 10 minutes. Shake basket halfway through.
4. Transfer cauliflower into the serving bowl. Add pine nuts and toss well.
5. Serve and enjoy.

Nutrition: Calories 139 Fat 13.1 g Carbohydrates 5.5 g Sugar 1.9 g Protein 2.7 g Cholesterol 0 mg

Thyme Sage Butternut Squash

Preparation Time:10 minutes

Cooking Time: 12 minutes

Servings:4

Ingredients:

- 2 lbs. butternut squash, cut into chunks
- 1 tsp fresh thyme, chopped
- 1 tbsp fresh sage, chopped
- 1 tbsp olive oil
- Pepper
- Salt

Directions:

1. Preheat the cosori air fryer to 390 F.
2. In a mixing bowl, toss butternut squash with thyme, sage, oil, pepper, and salt.
3. Add butternut squash into the air fryer basket and cook for 10 minutes. Shake basket well and cook for 2 minutes more.
4. Serve and enjoy.

Nutrition: Calories 50 Fat 3.8 g Carbohydrates 4.2 g Sugar 2.5 g Protein 1.4 g Cholesterol 0 mg

Grilled Cauliflower

Preparation Time:15 minutes

Cooking Time: 40 minutes

Servings: 4

Ingredients:

- 1 large head of cauliflower, leaves removed and stem trimmed
- Salt, as required
- 4 tablespoons unsalted butter
- ¼ cup hot sauce
- 1 tablespoon ketchup
- 1 tablespoon soy sauce
- 1/2 cup mayonnaise
- 2 tablespoons white miso
- 1 tablespoon fresh lemon juice
- 1/2 teaspoon ground black pepper
- 2 scallions, thinly sliced

Directions:

1. Sprinkle the cauliflower with salt evenly.
2. Arrange the cauliflower head in a large microwave-safe bowl.
3. With a plastic wrap, cover the bowl.

4. With a knife, pierce the plastic a few Times to vent.

5. Microwave on high for about 5 minutes.

6. Remove from the microwave and set aside to cool slightly.

7. In a small saucepan, add butter, hot sauce, ketchup and soy sauce over medium heat and cook for about 2-3 minutes, stirring occasionally.

8. Brush the cauliflower head with warm sauce evenly.

9. Place the water tray in the bottom of Power XL Smokeless Electric Grill.

10. Place about 2 cups of lukewarm water into the water tray.

11. Place the drip pan over water tray and then arrange the heating element.

12. Now, place the grilling pan over heating element.

13. Set the temperature settings according to manufacturer's Directions:

14. Cover the grill with lid and let it preheat.

15. After preheating, remove the lid and grease the grilling pan.

16. Place the cauliflower head over the grilling pan.
17. Cover with the lid and cook for about 10 minutes.
18. Turn the cauliflower over and brush with warm sauce.
19. Cover with the lid and cook for about 25 minutes, flipping and brushing with warm sauce after every 10 minutes.
20. In a bowl, place the mayonnaise, miso, lemon juice, and pepper and beat until smooth.
21. Spread the mayonnaise mixture onto a plate and arrange the cauliflower on top.

Nutrition: Calories 261 Total Fat 22 g Saturated Fat 8.9 g Cholesterol 38 mg Sodium 1300mg Total Carbs 15.1 g Fiber 2.5 g Sugar 5.4 g Protein 3.3 g

Stuffed Zucchini

Preparation Time: 20 minutes

Cooking Time: 24 minutes

Servings: 6

Ingredients:

- 3 medium zucchinis, sliced in half lengthwise
- 1 teaspoon vegetable oil
- 3 cup corn, cut off the cob
- 1 cup Parmesan cheese, shredded
- 2/3 cup sour cream
- ¼ teaspoon hot sauce
- Olive oil cooking spray

Directions:

1. Cut the ends off the zucchini and slice in half lengthwise.
2. Scoop out the pulp from each half of zucchini, leaving the shell.
3. For filling: in a large pan of boiling water, add the corn over medium heat and cook for about 5-7 minutes.
4. Drain the corn and set aside to cool.

5. In a large bowl, add corn, half of the parmesan cheese, sour cream and hot sauce and mix well.

6. Spray the zucchini shells with cooking spray evenly.

7. Place the water tray in the bottom of Power XL Smokeless Electric Grill.

8. Place about 2 cups of lukewarm water into the water tray.

9. Place the drip pan over water tray and then arrange the heating element.

10. Now, place the grilling pan over heating element.

11. Set the temperature settings according to manufacturer's Directions:

12. Cover the grill with lid and let it preheat.

13. After preheating, remove the lid and grease the grilling pan.

14. Place the zucchini halves over the grilling pan, flesh side down.

15. Cover with the lid and cook for about 8-10 minutes.

16. Remove the zucchini halves from grill.

17. Spoon filling into each zucchini half evenly and sprinkle with remaining parmesan cheese.
18. Place the zucchini halves over the grilling pan.
19. Cover with the lid and cook for about 8 minutes.
20. Serve hot.

Nutrition: Calories 198 Total Fat 10.8 g Saturated Fat 6 g Cholesterol 21 mg Sodium 293 mg Total Carbs 19.3 g Fiber 3.2 g Sugar 4.2 g Protein 9.6 g

Vinegar Veggies

Preparation Time: 15 minutes

Cooking Time: 10 minutes

Servings: 4

Ingredients:

- 3 golden beets, trimmed, peeled and sliced thinly
- 3 carrots, peeled and sliced lengthwise
- 1 cup zucchini, sliced
- 1 onion, sliced
- 1/2 cup yam, sliced thinly
- 2 tablespoon fresh rosemary
- 1 garlic clove, minced
- Salt and ground black pepper, as required
- 3 tablespoons vegetable oil
- 2 teaspoons balsamic vinegar

Directions:

1. Place all ingredients in a bowl and toss to coat well.
2. Refrigerate to marinate for at least 30 minutes.
3. Place the water tray in the bottom of Power XL Smokeless Electric Grill.

4. Place about 2 cups of lukewarm water into the water tray.
5. Place the drip pan over water tray and then arrange the heating element.
6. Now, place the grilling pan over heating element.
7. Plugin the Power XL Smokeless Electric Grill and press the 'Power' button to turn it on.
8. Then press 'Fan" button.
9. Set the temperature settings according to manufacturer's Directions:
10. Cover the grill with lid and let it preheat.
11. After preheating, remove the lid and grease the grilling pan.
12. Place the vegetables over the grilling pan.
13. Cover with the lid and cook for about 5 minutes per side.
14. Serve hot.

Nutrition: Calories 184 Total Fat 10.7 g Saturated Fat 2.2 g Cholesterol 0 mg Sodium 134 mg Total Carbs 21.5 g Fiber 4.9 g Sugar 10 g Protein 2.7 g

Garlicky Mixed Veggies

Preparation Time:15 minutes

Cooking Time: 8 minutes

Servings: 4

Ingredients:

- 1 bunch fresh asparagus, trimmed
- 6 ounces fresh mushrooms, halved
- 6 Campari tomatoes, halved
- 1 red onion, cut into 1-inch chunks
- 3 garlic cloves, minced
- 2 tablespoons olive oil
- Salt and ground black pepper, as required

Directions:

1. In a large bowl, add all ingredients and toss to coat well.
2. Place the water tray in the bottom of Power XL Smokeless Electric Grill.
3. Place about 2 cups of lukewarm water into the water tray.
4. Place the drip pan over water tray and then arrange the heating element.
5. Now, place the grilling pan over heating element.

6. Plugin the Power XL Smokeless Electric Grill and press the 'Power' button to turn it on.
7. Then press 'Fan" button.
8. Set the temperature settings according to manufacturer's Directions:
9. Cover the grill with lid and let it preheat.
10. After preheating, remove the lid and grease the grilling pan.
11. Place the vegetables over the grilling pan.
12. Cover with the lid and cook for about 8 minutes, flipping occasionally.

Nutrition: Calories 137 Total Fat 7.7 g Saturated Fat 1.1 g Cholesterol 0 mg Sodium 54 mg Total Carbs 15.6 g Fiber 5.6 g Sugar 8.9 g Protein 5.8 g

Mediterranean Veggies

Preparation Time:5 minutes

Cooking Time: 10 minutes

Servings: 4

Ingredients:

- 1 cup mixed bell peppers, chopped
- 1 cup eggplant, chopped
- 1 cup zucchini, chopped
- 1 cup mushrooms, chopped
- 1/2 cup onion, chopped
- 1/2 cup sun-dried tomato vinaigrette dressing

Directions:

1. In a large bowl, add all ingredients and toss to coat well.
2. Refrigerate to marinate for about 1 hour.
3. Place the water tray in the bottom of Power XL Smokeless Electric Grill.
4. Place about 2 cups of lukewarm water into the water tray.
5. Place the drip pan over water tray and then arrange the heating element.

6. Now, place the grilling pan over heating element.

7. Plugin the Power XL Smokeless Electric Grill and press the 'Power' button to turn it on.

8. Then press 'Fan" button.

9. Set the temperature settings according to manufacturer's Directions:

10. Cover the grill with lid and let it preheat.

11. After preheating, remove the lid and grease the grilling pan.

12. Place the vegetables over the grilling pan.

13. Cover with the lid and cook for about 8-10 minutes, flipping occasionally.

Nutrition: Calories 159 Total Fat 11.2 g Saturated Fat 2 g Cholesterol 0 mg Sodium 336 mg Total Carbs 12.3 g Fiber 1.9 g Sugar 9.5 g Protein 1.6 g

Marinated Veggie Skewers

Preparation Time:20 minutes

Cooking Time: 10 minutes

Servings: 4

Ingredients:

- For Marinade:
- 2 garlic cloves, minced
- 2 teaspoons fresh basil, minced
- 2 teaspoons fresh oregano, minced
- 1/2 teaspoon cayenne pepper
- Sea Salt and ground black pepper, as required
- 2 tablespoons fresh lemon juice
- 2 tablespoons olive oil
- For Veggies:
- 2 large zucchinis, cut into thick slices
- 8 large button mushrooms, quartered
- 1 yellow bell pepper, seeded and cubed
- 1 red bell pepper, seeded and cubed

Directions:

1. For marinade: in a large bowl, add all the ingredients and mix until well combined.
2. Add the vegetables and toss to coat well.

3. Cover and refrigerate to marinate for at least 6-8 hours.

4. Remove the vegetables from the bowl and thread onto pre-soaked wooden skewers.

5. Place the water tray in the bottom of Power XL Smokeless Electric Grill.

6. Place about 2 cups of lukewarm water into the water tray.

7. Place the drip pan over water tray and then arrange the heating element.

8. Now, place the grilling pan over heating element.

9. Plugin the Power XL Smokeless Electric Grill and press the 'Power' button to turn it on.

10. Then press 'Fan" button.

11. Set the temperature settings according to manufacturer's Directions: Cover the grill with lid and let it preheat.

12. After preheating, remove the lid and grease the grilling pan.

13. Place the skewers over the grilling pan. Cover with the lid and cook for about 8-10 minutes, flipping occasionally. Serve hot.

Nutrition: Calories 122 Total Fat 7.8 g Saturated Fat

1.2 g Cholesterol 0 mg Sodium 81 mg Total Carbs 12.7 g Fiber 3.5 g Sugar 6.8g Protein 4.3 g

Pineapple & Veggie Skewers

Preparation Time:20 minutes

Cooking Time: 15 minutes

Servings: 6

Ingredients:

- 1/3 cup olive oil
- 11/2 teaspoons dried basil
- ¾ teaspoon dried oregano
- Salt and ground black pepper, as required
- 2 zucchinis, cut into 1-inch slices
- 2 yellow squash, cut into 1-inch slices
- 1/2 pound whole fresh mushrooms
- 1 red bell pepper, cut into chunks
- 1 red onion, cut into chunks
- 12 cherry tomatoes
- 1 fresh pineapple, cut into chunks

Directions:

1. In a bowl, add oil, herbs, salt and black pepper and mix well.
2. Thread the veggies and pineapple onto pre-soaked wooden skewers.

3. Brush the veggies and pineapple with oil mixture evenly.
4. Place the water tray in the bottom of Power XL Smokeless Electric Grill.
5. Place about 2 cups of lukewarm water into the water tray.
6. Place the drip pan over water tray and then arrange the heating element.
7. Now, place the grilling pan over heating element.
8. Plugin the Power XL Smokeless Electric Grill and press the 'Power' button to turn it on.
9. Then press 'Fan" button.
10. Set the temperature settings according to manufacturer's Directions:
11. Cover the grill with lid and let it preheat.
12. After preheating, remove the lid and grease the grilling pan.
13. Place the skewers over the grilling pan.
14. Cover with the lid and cook for about 10-15 minutes, flipping occasionally.
15. Serve hot.

Nutrition: Calories 220 Total Fat 11.9 g Saturated Fat 1.7 g Cholesterol 0 mg Sodium 47 mg Total Carbs 30 g Fiber 5 g Sugar 20.4 g Protein 4.3 g

Buttered Corn

Preparation Time:10 minutes

Cooking Time: 20 minutes

Servings: 6

Ingredients:

- 6 fresh whole corn on the cob
- 1/2 cup butter, melted
- Salt, as required

Directions:

- Husk the corn and remove all the silk.
- Brush each corn with melted butter and sprinkle with salt.
- Place the water tray in the bottom of Power XL Smokeless Electric Grill.
- Place about 2 cups of lukewarm water into the water tray.
- Place the drip pan over water tray and then arrange the heating element.
- Now, place the grilling pan over heating element.
- Plugin the Power XL Smokeless Electric Grill and press the 'Power' button to turn it on.
- Then press 'Fan" button.

- Set the temperature settings according to manufacturer's Directions:
- Cover the grill with lid and let it preheat.
- After preheating, remove the lid and grease the grilling pan.
- Place the corn over the grilling pan.
- Cover with the lid and cook for about 20 minutes, rotating after every 5 minutes and brushing with butter once halfway through.
- Serve warm.

Nutrition: Calories 268 Total Fat 17.2 g Saturated Fat 10 g Cholesterol 41 mg Sodium 159 mg Total Carbs 29 g Fiber 4.2 g Sugar 5 g Protein 5.2 g